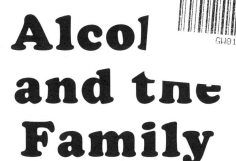

Alcohol and the Family

Three Sure Ways to Solve the Problem

Father Frank, C.SS.R.

LIGUORI
PUBLICATIONS

One Liguori Drive
Liguori, Missouri 63057
(314) 464-2500

Imprimi Potest:
Edmund T. Langton, C.SS.R.
Provincial, St. Louis Province
Redemptorist Fathers

Imprimatur:
+ John N. Wurm, S.T.D., Ph.D.
Vicar General, Archdiocese of St. Louis

ISBN 0-89243-086-9

Table of Contents

Prologue

This is no textbook. This is a pick-me-up-and-read-me-if-the-title-touches-you-any-way-at-all-from-any-angle-at-all. This little booklet is for anyone and everyone in the alcoholic family.

Don't be embarrassed. Thirty million people in the United States are sweating out alcoholism — in themselves and/or in their loved ones. People out there are dying tonight, going insane tonight, because of this disease.

We think you owe it to yourself and to them to read about it, to be able to talk about it and make sense, and not be satisfied to master a few "street names" and "street fears," as we might call many half-baked ideas of alcoholism.

For this reason, we include a "Glossary" on page 59.

We know that the fine professional volumes have already been written. We just want to set the stage for the characters to walk in on cue; and, believe it, the whole family has a part in this tragedy. Foremost among the actors and actresses will be the wives or husbands who cover up, protect, lie for, are ashamed for their partners. Finally, there is much to be said for the growing children, and to them.

So, this booklet cries out to you: READ ME! You have positively nothing to lose, and there really is hope. If you have to spell problem this way — A-L-C-O-H-O-L — then you may find a lot of happiness in these pages.

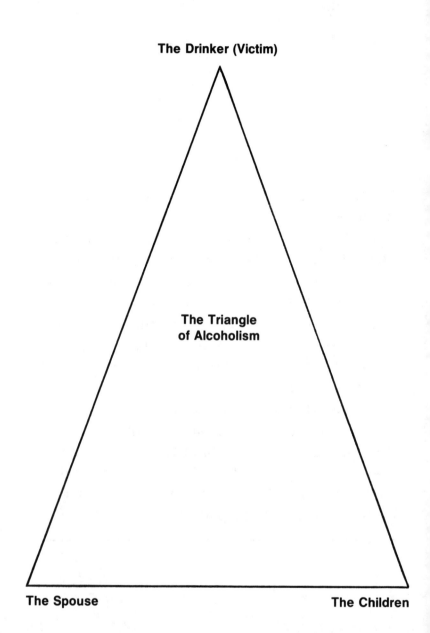

The Drinker (Victim)

The Triangle
of Alcoholism

The Spouse

The Children

CHAPTER 1
The Alcoholic

This is not a little old screaming crusade against the evils of alcohol. It is more a sweat meditation. I suppose a real practicing alcoholic has put this down by now. That is bad, because it means that such a one has not reached the knowing point, that place where one stands still long enough to hear one's entrails pleading: "Somebody help me! Whether I want it or not, somebody help me!"

The awful tragedy goes on. He does not know. She does not know. "Not me! It couldn't happen to me!" They have been struck with a corrosive disease. Their drinking and their lives are all out of shape. They want to drink like their friends, but they can't. What has happened to them, for God's sake?

At this point, the statistic sheet could be rolled out on the floor, but that never seems to get through to the guy or gal who is one of the numbers on the board. However, to get a few figures out of the way, let us say that there are about ten million alcoholics in the United States today, and each one affects approximately four in his family and sixteen in his circle — relatives, friends, employers, etc. Eighty thousand Americans die annually as the direct result of alcohol abuse.

As to the employer bit, the annual price tag on hangovers is over five billion dollars. Out of 50,000 highway deaths per year, alcohol plays a part in 28,000 of them. Fifty percent of the male admissions in mental hospitals, from ages 45 to 64, are listed under alcoholism. Some say that 50 percent of the juvenile delinquents have a background of parental alcoholism. But who counts? So, let us cut through and say right now that the best way, almost the only way, out of this hellish maze is Alcoholics Anonymous. Psychiatrists will not claim more than five percent success in treating alcoholics. Alcoholics Anonymous runs to 60 percent, 70 percent, and even 80 percent success. However, the point and purpose of this very unscientific booklet is to mull over and mumble over the here-and-now problem of the man or woman who is beginning to realize that he or she is no longer the "master of his destiny," as the poet says. Alcoholics

Anonymous puts it this way: "They cannot manage their lives anymore." They are compulsive drinkers. But you just hold on, brother, sister — help is on the way.

We might say here that there is quite a difference between a heavy drinker and an alcoholic, whom we might call a drinker with a problem. The first lad, the heavy drinker, may be disgusted with himself on Monday morning after the weekend binge. He gets up and goes to work, making and meaning great resolutions about the future. Physically and psychologically he is able to keep those resolutions, and does. He likes his beer a whole lot; but if the host does not have any, he will settle for a cola, and that is the end of it. There is no agony about it. There is no compulsion.

Not so the true alcoholic, the drinker with a problem. He gets up and, in many advanced cases, will feel that he needs a drink in order even to think about going to work that day. He may make a meaningless resolution; in fact, he may make three or four more resolutions later in the day. The picture is without humor. This man is a sick man. He has a disease. Dear God, help him call it by its name — alcoholism. It will be like tearing out his heart to admit it.

Note: It won't help much to argue about the hereditary aspect of alcoholism. Some say that there is no specific biological evidence of hereditary alcoholism. However, the National Council on Alcoholism states that where one parent is alcoholic, half the children have the sad chance of becoming alcoholic. Let us say that alcohol can be psychologically hereditary, in that there is a disorder in alcoholic families. There is a lack of good balance between love and discipline in dealing with the children. These problems make the children uptight and insecure. Hence we can find them prone (psychologically) to alcohol as a vent they see used more or less successfully at home by a parent or parents.

So, take a deep breath. God* knows all about you. If you have strayed from him, A.A. of itself cannot bring you back. Rather, it can quietly present to you the picture of how to come back. It cannot touch you in depth, however, unless you begin by taking your body to an A.A.

---

*Alcoholics Anonymous admits its own powerlessness over alcohol and, therefore, relies entirely on a "Higher Power." Most consider this Power to be God. At all events, it is a Power higher than the prostrate alcoholic or the bottle.

meeting. Your first great help along the road is simply (?) to admit that you cannot drink any more like your old buddies, that you really accept the fact that there is truly something wrong with you; alcohol has become a problem for you at one or more levels of your life. Something is nagging at you, and it is not a broken foot.

Alcoholics Anonymous is not going to challenge you. It will simply offer you a system that works, and then you can challenge the denying drunkard inside of you. Skirting around the scientific medical facts involved, let us simply say that the real alcoholic, somewhat like a diabetic, does not have the proper balance in his/her physical make-up. Whereas diabetics must have insulin or die, alcoholics cannot react normally to alcohol; and they will die (liver, heart) or go insane (brain) if they keep pouring alcohol into their defenseless systems. Alcoholics Anonymous is their way of fighting back and living — by complete abstinence. May the almighty God help you, as an alcoholic, realize that you are physically different from other men and other women, and you have to live that way, namely — without alcohol. Oh, that almighty first step of Alcoholics

Anonymous — "WE ADMITTED that we were powerless over alcohol and that our lives had become unmanageable." And it is so very hard to admit!

Let us now run a little movie, and you decide where and if you fit. We will not go into great details about the boners — the missed appointments, the bent fenders, etc. Furthermore, we will not talk about the morality, that is, the guilt or lack of guilt in your drinking. We don't blame a child for having diabetes. Much will depend on the stage of alcoholism at which this person is now existing. Again, good writers on the subject say that each drink must be judged on its own merits. However, there may well be guilt if, in a fairly sober moment, individuals truly realize that A.A. can help them and they positively refuse to investigate. So, we will simply call the morality debatable at this juncture: no sweeping recriminations and no sweeping absolutions. Let us see some pictures of that movie. Are you in it?

Loading up on liquor at home before going to a party is a very bad sign. Having a few ounces in the kitchen while making a new batch of drinks for company is a red, red signal of danger. So is gulping. (The alcoholic is a gulper with any liquid.) A late-night visit to the liquor store so as to be sure of a morning drink is also a flunking note. We may remark here that the nightly visitor still may have about 20 mystical hiding places around the house to make sure that the above problem will not lift its ugly head in the first place.

Just about this time somebody in the back row will shout out (or worse still, will quietly intimate) the completely false statement that one could not become an alcoholic if one drank only beer. Here are the facts:

1. Nobody really becomes an alcoholic. You have the "makings" or you don't.

2. One out of every fourteen *users* of this drug, ethyl alcohol, will show up on the chart as an alcoholic, whether through hard liquor, wine, or beer.

3. One can of beer equals one ounce of hard liquor, and equals four ounces of wine. Yes, a six-pack of beer equals at least six shots of hard liquor.

Blackouts are a turn in the road — for the worse. You may have been a perfect lady or gentleman at the party on the night before — danced sedately, conversed pleasantly — but the next morning you do not remember one thing that happened after the fourth (?) drink. Let's face it. As far as you know, you may have killed somebody with your car on the way home, and you do not know. *You do not know!* All you can do is read the papers, the death notices, or whatever. Your memory was there all right, but it was like a camera without film. Your blood cells were sick. And the other questions start raising their wet little heads. Did I insult a friend? Was I obscene in some story? Did I shock anyone? children?

Let the movie alone now, and tell me how this next sentence grabs you; it was written by an A.A. "Life went by me, lost in a whiskey haze; no love for God, no love for my wife, my children, my home."

You see, you have to stand still and peel off a few layers. Isn't your efficiency really going down? Are you getting pretty cranky around the house? Do you hate to hear people even bantering about alcohol? Is sleep difficult? Do you drink alone or with just anyone who provides companionship? Do you find yourself preferring taverns below your class? Do you need a belt of whiskey to start a job, to get over a funeral; or do you even let a few drinks take the place of a meal? These are red signals. Put very simply, alcoholism means that drink has become a problem in your life, doesn't it?

In the throes of his helplessness, the alcoholic will often turn to God, to prayer. Trusting in God is the heart of Alcoholics Anonymous — but it must be made very clear that religion cannot conquer alcoholism any more than it can conquer cancer. Surely there is a possibility of a miracle, but religion in A.A. does not bet on miracles; it quietly relies on the Twelve Steps within A.A. Never fear — you will find God waiting for you within those Twelve Steps, those twelve platforms of the Alcoholics Anonymous. Take great heart. God was there all the time, and you will learn to accept completely your alcoholic disease as right now God accepts you completely, just as you are. He will help you exactly where you are, and not where you should be.

I know that we are galloping along here in seven-league boots, jumping from peak to peak, and ignoring the valleys. That is exactly what we want to do. Alcoholics know all about valleys. They also know that up on the hills there are lots of men and women of A.A., sober for 10 to 20 to 30 years, who guarantee that there is a carload of happiness (no, change that to a carload of "reasonable contentment") as close to alcoholics as the phone book on the desk or in the kitchen. They will find Alcoholics Anonymous right where it belongs, listed alphabetically. For instance, here in St. Louis the address is in the business listings — 2683 Big Bend Boulevard. The telephone number is (314) 647-3677. In many large cities there is a 24-hour open line to A.A. In smaller towns you would be surprised to find out how much the chief of police knows about this matter and that he can give you proper direction and a lot of encouragement.

At any rate, in your A.A. phone call there will be just a pleasant hello from the other end — a brother, a sister alcoholic — with an offer to help if you wish and perhaps some small talk about the next meeting. Maybe it is tonight. You will be further told that, if you wish, you will be contacted by a member at a time that is agreeable to you. (Don't be too surprised if the fellow who turns up to take you to the meeting is the gentleman who has been ushering at your church every Sunday for the past eight years, and has been in Alcoholics Anonymous for the last nine years.)

You have to believe that if you are a true practicing alcoholic you will have a devil of a time reaching out for help, because you will want things the way you want them; and if they are not, you know how to use the bottle to make them come out your way. The sober truth is that society should be protected from such a one. To say it coldly, it is better to let A.A. do it for you — and for me.

The actual Alcoholics Anonymous meeting must be one of the rarest things upon this earth. It is a *real eyeopener* (for a change). The quiet, common bond between these people is a deeply peaceful thing, quite impossible to explain. Allegiances of color or creed or nationality simply fade away and no longer exist in the face of this other, this new bond. Ask any of those you meet there — butcher, baker, housewife, secretary, candlestick maker, lawyer, priest, judge — you name them! Sometimes one thinks that if this whole rather loveless world were alcoholic and became A.A. members, we would all at last be brothers and sisters in this deep caring bond. The last sentence is not in the least meant to be light. It is written in full conviction, unreal as it may seem. Alcoholics Anonymous kills the loner in us all, and that word "loner" is a heartbreak to an alcoholic. Alcoholics have been there, in Lonesville, so often. How good it is now to find others exactly like themselves. They can hardly believe it. They are home at last! And the door is wide open! Dear God, it feels good to have no one looking down on you, blaming you. These people have been through it all! They know what it means not to be able to remember, not to know why your best friends have asked you not to come back.

About the meeting. The A.A. is not a secret society. In fact, its very outwardness and simplicity might leave your mouth positively gaping. It is just a bunch of guys and gals around a table, or perhaps 10 tables, drinking coffee and maybe smoking and talking. Talking about what? "My little Shirley lost two of her baby teeth last week." "My mother died last week, and I had a hard time passing by the neighborhood bar that night. But I sweated it out." "Good boy, Joe," someone says. He means it, and we all smile and happily grunt congratulations.

The captain of each table is somebody, anybody, who has been a member for a certain period and can conduct a discussion. Often the choice is made something like this: "Fred (or Linda), will you take table three tonight? They want to talk about the A.A. fourth step." So the tables start. Someone will read the step or steps about which the discussion will be involved. The members may take turns right down the line; the system varies very little around the world. Their talk might run like this: "This step was hard for me, but I think I am catching on." Others might tell how they had at last seen through the fourth step or the seventh step or whatever. Sometimes a special speaker appears. He will be an A.A. member, of course (and often may hit the professional circuit for the cause), and this usually turns out to be quite a treat. The man or woman is a professional!

THE TWELVE STEPS

These Steps have been mentioned quite often, so perhaps this is a good place to set them down.

We:
1. Admitted that we were powerless over alcohol — that our lives had become unmanageable.

2. Came to believe that a Power greater than ourselves could restore us to sanity.

3. Made a decision to turn our will and our lives over to the care of God as we understood him.

4. Made a searching and fearless moral inventory of ourselves.

5. Admitted to God, to ourselves, and to another human being the exact nature of our wrongs.

6. Were entirely ready to have God remove all these defects of character.

7. Humbly asked him to remove our shortcomings.

8. Made a list of all the persons we had harmed, and became willing to make amends to them all.

9. Made direct amends to such people wherever possible, except when to do so would injure them or others.

10. Continued to take personal inventory, and when we were wrong, promptly admitted it.

11. Sought through prayer and meditation to improve our conscious contact with God as we understood him, praying only for knowledge of his will for us and the power to carry that out.

12. Tried to carry this message to alcoholics and to practice these principles in all our affairs.

Dear friend, you may perhaps look at those Twelve Steps and shake your head, gratefully thinking that you do not have to go through all that. Don't you? Then let's run through another list of twelve. If you have any one of the following problems or factors, *you are an alcoholic!*

1. Do you drink to calm nerves or sedate yourself?
2. Does your irritability increase while you are drinking?
3. Do you frequently drink until quite drunk?
4. Do you have special hiding places for liquor?
5. Are you steadily increasing your intake of alcohol?
6. Do you lie about your drinking?
7. Do you have a drink the first thing in the morning?
8. Do you miss work, shirk duties because of drinking?
9. Do you neglect your family?
10. Are you having periods of memory failure?
11. Have you been hospitalized for drinking?
12. Have you lost your job because of alcohol?

* * * * * *

Books have been written on the solid spirituality and effectiveness of the Twelve Steps: twelve ways back to God and sobriety or, better perhaps, to sobriety and God. Sobriety first: you don't want to be drunk when you are praying.

It is very surprising to discover that only in the first two of the Twelve Steps is alcohol mentioned. The others are all about you and your God and your fellow alcoholic sufferer. Everything is right there in the Steps. It is worth everything that you hold dear to know them and to try to live them — your salvation in one dozen little sentences. Easy does it, though. One step at a time, please. You have had enough tension! Just let go and let God. Your new A.A. friends will help. They hope you will ask.

What is the secret of this success? The jury system! There is no prosecutor, defender or judge. The jury is made up of peers, that is, equals, and they chew over the problem and hand each other the knowledge and the decisions and the strength and the consolation that each one needs. Let's put it this way — if ten prisoners were to be freed and if statistics would tell us that three would return to prison, who would best be able to tell us which three would be back? Right! The prisoners themselves. The jury has chewed it and the jury knows. They lived with it. They can set you straight, can point out the pitfalls of resentment and fear.

Here one person affirms another. We call him or her the sponsor, your sponsor. This person will be very important in your new life. We are all grateful to these sponsors because they enlightened us, lifted us over the early going. Books are written about them, and you will learn from them at first hand.

So, come on in from the cold. You will find that sobriety is a very sacred word to these people. The alcoholic will seldom say: "I have been dry seven years," but, rather, "I have kept (have had) my sobriety for seven years." "My" sobriety — the dearest of possessions.

Alcoholics are not hilarious over their sobriety. They quietly realize that they have a 24-hour-a-day problem and that they must be satisfied with being "reasonably content." They know that their greatest mistake would be to think that they can ever in this earthly life return to social drinking, return to alcohol.

During their alcoholic career they ran into many problems because they were loners. And when it comes to the great American custom of being handed a drink on entering just about any house, they must become loners all over again. But they do it. They have looked hard at their fears and alibis, their resentments, their pride, their self-pity; and they have thrown away the values on which these were based. They have an A.A. meeting tonight at 7:30. They will meet again the group they have been loyal to once more by refusing that drink, and loyal once more to their God, and loyal once more to themselves.

May we close this chapter in the way that each meeting of Alcoholics Anonymous closes — with the "Our Father." Let us all say that great prayer right now, asking the Highest Power of all to shed light and strength upon the wandering ones out there who must find A.A. or death or insanity. Because that's the way it is. There is no other way. And you can't just let it go on, can you? Will you? Reach for the phone, friend.

Our Father, who art in heaven, hallowed be thy name; thy kingdom come; thy will be done on earth as it is in heaven. Give us this day our daily bread; and forgive us our trespasses as we forgive those who trespass against us; and lead us not into temptation, but deliver us from evil. Amen.

CHAPTER 2
The Spouse

Lots of shutters have been thrown back, curtains raised, and the United States and other countries have had a well-advertised look into the alcoholics living room, kitchen, baby crib, and any other space where a bottle might be stashed. No doubt about it, a lot of good has been done. Penetrating articles have been written and detoxification headquarters and halfway houses and convalescent homes have been allowed to come up out of the basement. And, with vigor, well-known people of stage and screen, business and politics, alcoholics all, have told their stories and encouraged other alcoholics to come in out of the cold. Finally, and denoting the new thinking, alcohol bottles may soon have to carry a caution, warning of the hazards of this chemical called alcohol.

And now let's reach out a hand to the nonalcoholic spouse who has just about been sunk beneath the waves of guilt, shame, endless advice, threats, and hopeless heart-break. Note: We should make it clear at once that we realize that the wife may be the alcoholic in many cases, and the husband is the one going through all the agony of being married to a practicing alcoholic. However, for the greater part in these lines, we want to speak to you, the wife of the alcoholic.

We often find that your own decent pride as a human being and, above all, as a homemaker is the very thing that makes you so vulnerable. Who wants to admit failure? You feel like a hypocrite because you try to carry on as though nothing were wrong, while all the time you can almost see the word "failure" painted right across the front of your house. Your alcoholic husband is not quite satisfied with liquor; he is also, if we may use a less than pretty com-parison, blindly siphoning the blood from your heart. Perhaps now and then he recognizes what he is doing, but alcohol will quickly drown any remorse.

What must be made very clear is that this problem is not going to take care of itself. It will not just go away. Your alcoholic spouse has a progressive disease; he is going down and tak-ing you and your family with him. *If you think that the alcoholic cannot be helped until he wants to be helped, you had better start getting completely rid of any such idea.* The opposite is true; he won't stop drinking until he is forced to stop. The shrewdness with which he escapes any confrontation on this matter is almost diabolic. As Dr. David Youel, educational program coordinator for internal medicine at Western Michigan University in Kalamazoo, puts it: "A high recovery rate is possible only where the alcoholic can be helped *before* he wants to be helped. The boss, the labor union, the family — somebody has to box him in!"

His disease is called alcoholism. Yours, dear nonalcoholic, is called neuroticism. You cannot keep up this lying to friends, lying to the children, lying even to yourself. Let us say right here that if you do conquer this problem, and you can, it will hardly be without the help of others who are in the identical situation, the same boat, that you are in, mainly, the people of Al-Anon. We will later explain this group. Right now we want to get the picture straight.

Earlier, we called the nonalcoholic spouse helpless. We would like to give an example. Alcoholics, as we said, are very crafty people. Your husband must quickly close off any approach that might lead to his giving up alcohol. He comes on to the stage in the roles of different characters and also brings in a new hat each time for you to wear. One favorite costume is that of "persecutor." Of course, the nonalcoholic person is the "persecutor." In truth, the alcoholic is afraid that you may get fed up with his bullying and leave him. So, if you even open your mouth in protest, you are a "persecutor," and can put on that hat.

Mainly, however, it is because his self-image is so low that he unconsciously looks for your insults and protests as confirmation of his inferior feeling that he is a worthless wretch. And soon he needs you back in your "rescuer" hat to pick him up and go on with this game of cover up.

Or you may begin to initiate little games of your own, as you see yourself backed into one of the crazy corners of this crazy game. It would run this way: "I just won't prepare any dinner tonight because he will just come home too late, and/or drunk." Then you remember you have to cook for the children! You know that they are beginning to play you against your husband and him against you. You know they are becoming self-styled martyrs, paid off by everyone with pity, compassion, and even a few bucks. The youngsters know what they are doing and feel cheap about it, but they still go out to get away from the hell. How do you tell them to stay home and study in a house like this?

So what are you to do now? You join Al-Anon (the name is a shortening of Alcoholics Anonymous). It is just about your only chance, but a beautiful chance it is. The Al-Anon is basically a group of people who are married to alcoholics, although other interested people are also welcome. We might say that Al-Anon is a family group that works *around,* not *on* or *at,* the alcoholic. These people have meetings much like the A.A. meetings of the Alcoholics Anonymous. They use the principal steps and traditions of the Alcoholics Anonymous. They seek courage and structure and companionship despite the condition of their spouses. One way of getting in touch with them is to take the phone book, find those words "Alcoholics Anonymous," and dial that number. Ask for information about the Al-Anon group and their meetings. Believe me, the one on the other end of the line will be a person who has been through it all and is ready to go right down the line with you. You will be told the addresses of one or more Al-Anon meeting places near you. If you live in a small town and would rather attend meetings somewhere else, a good professional police chief may be the best one for you to approach. At all events, when you make the phone call, you will be informed that an Al-Anon member will call on you, even tonight if you wish, and take you to your first meeting, smoothing the way for you. Trust these people! They will help you.

Please understand that I am talking about a whole new life for you, an organized structure that does not wait until your husband wants to be helped but, instead, takes the first long beautiful stride toward finding a positive way of life for you. If your husband straightens out as a fringe benefit of your new life with the Al-Anon group, fine and dandy. If he does not, well then, that is his problem, not yours. That may sound harsh, but, honey, this is a harsh disease. There is no pill for this one! On the contrary, your husband is a sick man who insists on what is evidently the wrong medicine for him — alcohol. You have a life to live, perhaps a family of children to protect, and Al-Anon is going to show you how to do it. Your life of appeasing your spouse one day and nagging at him the next is over, if you are willing to follow the new rules.

One remark here: If there is any sin involved in all this, I would say that it is rather on the side of babying him and taking up for him, etc., than on the side of "being mean" and causing him to face up to his crisis.

About that word "crisis," it means what Dr. Youel called "boxing him in." Don't stand there while he goes all the way down and destroys himself on the rocks. The professionals in alcoholism talk about creating a crisis, such as one that was set off when the teen-age people of a certain home simply had had it and screamed out that they would never again bring their friends home to this drunkard, now awakening amidst his alcoholic vapors on the living room couch — their father! A shock like that — from one's own children — has been well called "confrontation," and at times it has been enough of a crisis to start the alcoholic up the dry side of the hill. Again, it is called "tough love," which is certainly a good name for it, because true love cannot stand there and watch the beloved die. *True love must turn into tough love.* Be as tough as it takes to get his attention — Roman candles, neon lights, the whole thing!

These crises must be so structured that the alcoholic can get the total picture, can be fully confronted. Some way, somehow, the alcoholic must find it more painful to drink than not to drink. Al-Anon will teach you these things.

Speaking of Al-Anon, let me quote one of them. She, an "almost suicide," turned to God (after much stomach pumping for pills) and could finally write: "I realize now that I am powerless. I trust God and on my part I take care of myself and try to improve myself, my children, my family. Al-Anon is my food and air. I am so much better off than my poor husband. He is the one who is missing so much, not I. He does not have the pleasure of seeing the children grow, and all it means. I have a job to do here, and I cannot do it as a self-pitying neurotic. Al-Anon showed me that its purpose was not to work miracles, but to instruct me to help myself. Now I clean the house, have my hair done, read a good book, sew — all this, not with a vengeance but with a peaceful plan. I have a beautiful new life. I am aware of people and have the desire to help them find the serenity I have today. My greatest compliment came from my 14-year-old son, who said one day, 'Mom, how come you are so happy and Dad is still drinking?' "

WHAT ABOUT DIVORCE?

Professionals in alcoholic counseling are properly slow to talk about divorce. Divorce means that things have gone along too far and now the crash is so bad that the last action of divorce must be taken. If it must be, then so be it. If we are talking about a husband and wife and three children, then the counselor can hardly be expected to put the one alcoholic person before the other four suffering persons. Of course, if your husband is a positive physical or spiritual danger to you or the children, then action must be taken, but he must not be allowed to put the decision and its effects on your shoulders.

We firmly pray and hope that no one reading these lines is simply letting everything slide downhill until there is nothing left but a divorce court. That is why we beg you, divorced or not, to get in touch with Al-Anon today.

Father James Schwertley, a practiced, knowledgeable person in the alcoholic divorce problem, has this to say: "Many alcoholics' wives, especially Catholics, agonize over whether to file for divorce or not. They ask such questions as: Will it scare the husband into getting some help for himself? Will it ruin him completely? Will I still be able to go to the sacraments? Is alcoholism a basis for a divorce in the Church's view? What legal protections do I have if there is threat of violence or withdrawal of financial support? How will the children be affected? How will I be affected?" To quote Father Schwertley again: "No reputable counselor will tell an alcoholic's wife that she should or should not get a divorce. That's HER decision. Every alcoholic puts different pressures on the wife, and every wife has different levels of tolerance. Only the affected individual can decide accurately, but a counselor can help examine the alternatives objectively and knowledgeably so that a clearer decision can be reached.

"There are certain guidelines that can provide a framework for decision by an alcoholic's wife (or husband). These have such validity that they might be called 'The Ten Commandments for Alcoholics' Wives.' Here they are.

1. Alcoholism is grounds for divorce in the view of the Church because God does not require you to live in inhuman conditions that you

did not cause. Note: Work with your pastor or associate pastor throughout this problem. They will advise you.

2. It is vital to file for divorce only when CONVINCED that you cannot live like that any longer and have nothing to lose.

3. Divorce should be a last resort, not only because of the importance of marriage but also because there are other things you can do first — such as Al-Anon and counseling — to create a crisis in the drinker's life.

4. Threatening divorce and then backing down weakens your position.

5. Going through with or filing for divorce JUST to try to scare the man into seeking help is not a good decision since it may not work.

6. Staying together 'for the sake of the children' is useless because children are better off with one parent who is relatively stable than with two parents in conflict.

7. People who urge you to get a divorce or tell you to 'hang on no matter what' are unfairly trying to run your life, however well-meaning they are.

8. If the alcoholic threatens violence or withholds support money, you have legal recourse available.

9. Being paralyzed by the thought of how you might get along alone for the rest of your life is an unreasonable fear, because you live your life in 24-hour sections, not 50-year chunks.

10. Your husband's threats of what might happen to him if you divorce him are groundless, because that's his problem, not yours."

Perhaps you wonder why we have hardly spoken of God or, as we call the Supreme Being in Alcoholics Anonymous, the Higher Power. We think it is better for you yourself to seek God quietly in the Al-Anons rather than have us preach to you. You will find God waiting there for you. Really, just the first two steps of A.A. have to do with alcohol. The remaining steps are primarily about God, believing in him, trusting in him, praying to him, and living with him. Then the final steps are given over to the love of our neighbor, the asking of forgiveness, the restoring of property and reputations, the willingness to go out of our way to help other alcoholics or spouses who are moving toward trouble, moving even toward despair.

It might be profitable now to take one last look at that idea of "cover-up." Believe the professionals again, believe those who have gone through this, that the alcoholic cannot even admit to the simple common denominator of all alcoholics, namely, that he has a problem due to alcohol. He hates to hear even the slightest joke about alcoholism. He cannot stand it being discussed. How is it that the person who has cancer or, let us say, heart disease has no such terrible obsession to cover up his affliction? On the other side of the coin, the practicing alcoholic will often deny to his dying breath that he has a drinking problem; imagine that! not even a problem! The answer is that, being obsessed with the drug alcohol, he cannot face the monumental decision to quit pouring it into his system. Also, of course, there is a public stigma attached to the illness, as there is with, let us say mental illness. This increases the tendency to deny it even in the face of overwhelming evidence that it is present.

Then everybody gets into the cover-up game, the spouse, the boss, the friends, the doctor, the boys at the bar, even the children. His best friends won't talk about it, even when it has advanced to an unbelievable stage. Why this? Well for one thing there is the ignorance of the real nature and price of alcoholism. That is why we so deeply hope that you will get in touch with Al-Anon. There you can at least get the picture straight. If your husband does make a comeback or even if he is still addicted and dependent on chemicals (and alcohol is one of them), it is important for you to know the structure and nature of alcoholism, instead of having mastered some few "street names" and "street fears" about it.

Furthermore, your attendance at Al-Anon will help you see how you have changed, and that you would otherwise not be able to understand how it was with him. You must learn to watch closely for the signs that tell you he is on the way back. He is trying to become healed and needs you as his helpmate — as you promised at the altar many years ago — not an amazon bearing down on him and reminding him what he has been the last 10 years, the awful thing he has been for the last 12 years, or whatever.

At no place in these lines do we want to be dishonest and not recognize in all of us a fear of confronting anybody on this sensitive issue. Again, here is where only "tough love" can help.

Dear friend, dear seeking friend, we cannot

promise you some kind of hilarious happiness. Alcoholics Anonymous talks only about being "reasonably content." Please God, may you find it — just one telephone call away.

CHAPTER 3
The Children

Some time ago there was a national meeting of Alcoholics Anonymous in Phoenix, Arizona, during which this writer was deeply moved by a young high-school senior boy who spoke his piece.

He was the son of an alcoholic mother. He did not talk much about how things were at home, about walking through rooms of soiled clothes, about watching his kid sisters and brothers going off to school with half a cold breakfast in them. Rather, he talked about the decision he had to make for his own peace of mind, and how he had to outthink the daily manipulations of his alcoholic parent in order to carry out this decision.

When he finished, a young 15-year-old girl rose to talk to us about her life with an alcoholic father. There was no trauma in this young lady, just plenty of poise. She could tell it the way it was.

These young people did not simply talk to us; they sang to us, as it were. We really began to see where it is with the young Alateens. We began to understand, too, in a little way, what it must be like for an even smaller child in an alcoholic home, a child who does not know whether the next moment will bring a kiss or a kick, depending on how the diseased parent is feeling at that moment.

Speaking again about (and for) this younger child, we must all realize that, due to parental alcoholism, the youngster finds himself or herself in a very unreal world that he or she simply cannot cope with. There is an endless need to take up for mother or father, whichever seems to offer the greatest security to the child at that moment. How shall that youngster ever live on terms of intimate trust with anyone, including a spouse someday? What a havoc of lives is to be laid at the door of the alcoholic parent — the door of that shambles called alcoholism. Well, there is no use in going into all that right now. Alcoholics Anonymous deals with the present 24 hours.

To return to the group at Phoenix, there is this to be said, and it is a very important thing indeed: These young people have actually found their way through the help of the Alateen group. Their meetings are not a crying session; instead, the members frankly talk over their problems with other teen-age people. They recognize the fact that they too have the problem, obligation, and privilege of helping *themselves.* Helping their alcoholic parent might be a fringe benefit, but never the target.

These young people impressed me, I say it again, because they simply knew where they were going and how to get there. One of them actually announced that he knew he could get away with anything short of murder and blame the whole thing on his parents, blame the whole thing on the hopeless destruction of his home life, and go on swinging from there. Alateen, he said, had moved in on him and offered instead a sense of responsibility, a soul-shaking conviction that he must *first* do the best that he could to make *his* life a success. He accepted the basic, well-tested approach of Alcoholics Anonymous:

God, grant me the serenity to accept
the things I cannot change,
the courage to change the things I can,
and the wisdom to know the difference.

Before we comment on what you should seek in your Alateen meetings, let us take this last look at some of the dos and don'ts for a young man or woman in an alcoholic household. After all, the very word Alateen means a teen-ager who is involved in the problem of alcoholism. (In the following paragraphs we designate the alcoholic person as a man, but it may very well be a woman.)

Be kind; the alcoholic victim already has a sense of guilt. He already has a low enough image of himself. Your parent knows that something inside him is all wrong; he just has not been able to come to terms with it — yet — alone. Please God, his sobriety may finally be *the* fringe benefit in a house where Al-Anons and Alateens live their own lives by A.A. principles and steps as developed and individualized by the parent group.

Meanwhile, do not protect him; that is not kindness for him. It is a miserable tragedy when the family will not admit that the father is a drunkard and will not treat him like the diseased alcoholic that he is until it is too late. On the contrary, you should try to make his drinking cause him more pain and problems than non-drinking does. For example, let him use his own money to pay the baby-sitter while the wife and other children take nights out socially, ignoring him except to indicate that his irresponsible drinking is making him shell out for the baby-sitter. All because he cannot be trusted to take care of the child! Make drinking as painful to him as possible. He knows — we know — that you are not really ignoring him. Yes, let his alcoholism know pain. Actually, this is a kindness.

Don't shelter him from a crisis. Instead, let it happen. Confront him with the day, the hour, the place. Don't stand there and let him go down the drain. True love is tough love. The principles are the same as in chapter one.

In a sense, the Alateen does not have certain advantages of the Al-Anon. For one thing the latter has the better part emotionally, because she is involved in the undertones of man-woman love, whereas the child is not. Again, the mother's circle of adult friends, her ability to contact them officially would be advantages not present to the young person. Far from discouraging the youngsters, however, this should impel them to go deeper into Alateen, to exchange ideas and solutions, and actively to keep each meeting very much alive and exciting until it is milked dry of every last drop of know-how and motivation.

Do not ever feel alone, dear young man or woman. There are about 13 million teen-agers in the United States trying to face and solve this same problem. What should you do? Find a corner and cry out your lives in self-pity? Nuts! The world belongs to the young! Go get it! Your new world is waiting in Alateen!

The first thing that Alateen insists that you do is to clear the ground of misunderstanding. This means that you are to realize that the alcoholic parent is not a spineless, weak-willed, irresponsible, evil old monster. He is sick. She is sick. They hate the disease and are in agony because they know it looks like they do not love you. God has told you, it is true, to honor your parents, so you must steadily ask that same God to help you understand, help you see through that parent's messy appearance, the confused speech, the endless lies and contradictions, and, beneath it all, to find a sick person who hopes you will somehow understand.

Next, Alateen will ask you to grow up, real big and real fast, because you have a real big, grown-up problem; and, as the fellow says: "Here is where we separate the men from the boys and the women from the girls." What we are really saying is that we hope you at once join the Alateens and begin to let the Twelve Steps move in on your life. Would you be able to phone them right now? You need only look up Alcoholics Anonymous in the phone book, and there will be someone on the other end of the line who will very kindly explain and answer any doubt or question you might have. Please do. Your whole future may be that telephone, right now.

Alateen will ask you to look at that life of yours, not at the life of your alcoholic parent. You will gradually realize that you can blame everything from A to Z on that parent, but it will not do you one bit of good as a person who wants to grow. Maybe your father (or mother) cannot be changed, but *you* can. *Your* speech, *your* habits, *your* dress are the things that count. You must succeed in studies because *you* are *you.* You must go first-class until hell freezes over! Get out there and sympathize with everybody's faults and problems except your own; don't waste time and tears on those. These may seem like very high ideals and fierce demands, but, dear God, isn't that what youth is for? To challenge life, to look the bad breaks in the eye and to go on?

Please, I repeat, please, do not feel and act like a persecuted martyr, or you will miss the whole point of growth and never become the wonderful person that you could be.

It is only fair to admit that the Alateens may have real difficulty in finding a time and a place for their meetings during the school year. Here in the United States there are five nights a week in which there is homework. Again, Friday night seems to be given over to a show and some relaxation, and Saturday night is quite often involved in dates. So, to be realistic, we have to break through someplace in there, and the normal suggestion is that the Alateens have their group meeting on the same night as A.A. or Al-Anon and in the same building. Even though this system would bite into some study time or demand some kind of car pool, the meetings do not last all that long, and certainly what is involved here is a lot more important than the next day's studies. We are dealing with a human being's life and a family's very existence.

None of this is easy. But you do have new lives at your fingertips, and not just your own life. There is also the one who gave you life and love as long as he could, as long as she could.

Now, please God, you can give back life, give back love. They sit there, hoping that you will start with *you;* because that's the way it is, and you can't just let it go on, can you? Will you?

The Triangles of Alcoholism

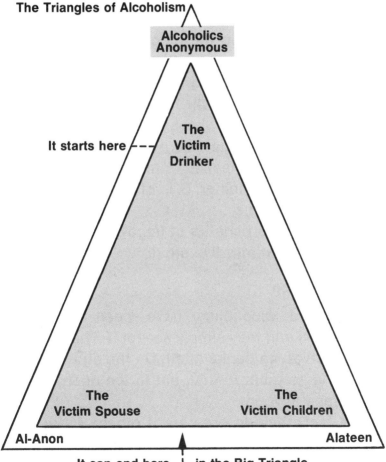

Alcoholics Anonymous

It starts here - -

The Victim Drinker

The Victim Spouse

The Victim Children

Al-Anon

Alateen

It can end here . ! . in the Big Triangle.

CHAPTER 4
What's It Like to Come Back?

Having examined the programs designed to help the alcoholic himself/herself, the spouse of the alcoholic, and the children of the alcoholic, we like to ask: "What's it like to come back?" Only those who have come back can truly answer this question. Here then are some of their answers gleaned from a research made by Rev. Joseph Fichter, S.J., of Loyola University in New Orleans.

Roughly, the benefits of (recovered) sobriety can be divided into five areas.

General Area

Arrested alcoholics have been given a diagnosis and they simply accept it. There is no mad denial, no denial at all. On the other hand, there is no guilt. It is all out in the open. They can face anybody.

In fact, they do not care if others do know. There is no need or room for that low self-esteem image. To arrive at this attitude is a thing of joy.

Deep in their minds they know they do not have to drink. No guilt, no denial — they look it in the eye and they do not have to drink.

They see where A.A. wants to lead them, and they willingly subject themselves to its guidance, to its indoctrination.

They have become comfortable in their participation in Alcoholics Anonymous. They realize they are talking commitment, and they are glad of it.

Social Area

There is now a sense of self-worth, and that was the precious gem that they had lost. Formerly, they were called lots of names, and often they could only bow their heads to accusations and recriminations. Not always remembering whether they had done this or that, they could not risk denial and take the chance of being confronted with dates and times. Now, respected once again, their advice is often sought.

Through the grace of God, their Higher Power, they look back at the field of battle where they have won their spurs. One very important thing they discovered was that old friends, etc. were not waiting in line to slap them on the back and cry out endless congratulations. The simple fact is that the ordinary person looks upon the ability to drink alcohol properly as the *ordinary* way of life and merits no applause. That is where A.A. comes in so beautifully; one member can quietly tell another member of his/her little victory and then they both share. This is growth.

They begin to look people in the eye. The Twelve Steps have acted as a catharsis; after admitting the problem, the alcoholic begins and continues a program of cleansing and forgiving and restoring. Because there is no guilt and no denial in his eyes, others have to take him at his here-and-now face value, and the new A.A. person is not afraid of that any longer. There was a pastor who discovered that he was an alcoholic and, finally, went away to take the course, as we may call it. When he had completed the schedule, he came back to his church and shook hands on a Sunday morning with all his people as they came through the doorway. Many of them cried silently, joyfully, as they walked up the aisle — and he was crying too.

We repeat, however, that alcoholic persons know that they will not always be received socially with a banner that cries out "Welcome Home — All Is Forgiven!" In the first place, "arrested" alcoholics do not really need any banners. Remember — no denial, no guilt. They are willing to let you take them as they are, so long as you make some little effort to find out who they *really* are *now.* The alcoholics know that they have to keep getting behind the eyeballs of the other person, getting into the memory of the other person who knew them when, and they understand if there is some reluctance to renew a broken friendship. They realize that they have to show proof that they are quite different persons; but all the while there is the deep-down happiness that no one can take from them, namely, that they know they have begun, at last, to turn *out* to others, not *in* to themselves — because that's where the unresolved battle was before they conceded victory to the bottle. "You win, bottle. I can't fight you any more. Good-bye. It is your battle field, or should I say 'bottle' field. Anyway, I surrender. I am going home, and you cannot come."

Work Area

They want to try their hand at their work again. It is not a time for talk, they know, but a time for achievement. However, they are not set only upon making good in the eyes of others; they are very interested in making good in their own eyes. Instead of every action being alcohol oriented, or else without value for them, now new horizons and purpose are in sight. Instead of frustration, there is a desire to tackle new dawns, because so many were clouded over in the past.

No longer are there authority or resentment hang-ups. In the past, resentment was the great alibi, and now they want to make it without alibis. There is tone in this man's, in this woman's spirit.

They now know how to pace their work, leaving room for the spiritual side of their lives, not running out of gas by 9:00 p.m. (Some of them remember from the past that liquor became their crutch at that hour — when they could not slow down after a slap-dash, chaotic day.)

They take time off now and embrace their vacations without any sense of guilt. Formerly, their work had been so shabby that they felt they did not deserve a vacation. And when they left, everyone knew that theirs would be a very wet vacation, even though they went to a dry climate. But now they are ready and able to show the world that they will not make a binge out of their days away, and so there is no feeling of guilt as they go off to relax.

They find their work satisfying and challenging. They regret all the time that was lost, and they are fulfilled as they accept the challenge of today and all the todays that God will give them.

Psychological Area

They are less tense now, less nervous, less worried; they let their world, at work or at home, see a true and full performance. They know, as we said before, that there will be no great slaps on the back. "Why celebrate?" others will think. "We have been on the ball all these years, and you have been operating at about a 12 percent efficiency." The A.A.'s humbly accept this and do not let it throw them. Humility is the heart of the matter now. Humility means knowing who we are and acting like it.

They have learned to trust in their Higher Power, their God, and are therefore less tempted to run to the bottle, that everlasting crutch, to overcome depression. In fact, they are even optimistic. The professional in them wants to get back to work.

Physical Area

They are overwhelmed at that beautiful human sensation called "feeling good." And, because they feel good, they reach out for a health program, so that the good feeling will blossom.

Epilogue

And now, the good news!

How can you tell when you are winning? You find yourself accepting responsibility for your own life — paying bills, taking an interest in your job and family situations and life in general. You find yourself increasingly more cheerful in dealing with people. You are able to postpone present gratification for greater goals without sulking or griping. You are beginning to do away with unreasonable perfectionism and expectations. You are willing to admit a fault when you are wrong.

And most important, you find yourself attending at least one or two Alcoholics Anonymous meetings a week, along with a sincere effort to help other alcoholics; and, down deep, you begin to want to help others, caught with this disease, find a beautiful new life.

Surely we all remember that mean old miser named Scrooge, whom Dickens gave us in his immortal **A Christmas Carol.** Oh, how we agonized with him when in his dreams he was confronted with his evil ways, his selfishness, his meanness. Finally, Scrooge was given a view of his dated headstone in the cemetery. And then — he woke up gloriously from his dream and found he was alive. Oh, how he ran and jumped and danced in pure joy at knowing it was not too late. And we awakened mortals rejoice with him as we shyly rub one foot against the other to be sure that we, too, are on top of the turf.

All that can be yours, too, fellow alcoholic. Wake up! The dream is over. You are alive! And here we are to help you, to share with you the blessings of life. So, let's all say together the great prayer that Alcoholics Anonymous will say today and tonight and all the 24 hours that our Father in heaven gives us.

Our Father, who art in heaven, hallowed be thy name; thy kingdom come; thy will be done on earth as it is in heaven. Give us this day our daily bread; and forgive us our trespasses as we forgive those who trespass against us; and lead us not into temptation, but deliver us from evil. Amen.

And as we close out each A.A. meeting:

For thine is the kingdom, and the power, and the glory, forever and ever. Amen.

Glossary

Disease of Alcoholism

There are approximately 150 definitions of alcoholism. We could group these definitions according to the way the alcoholic is affected by this disease, namely, spiritually, psychologically, physically, and socially. As you see, the person is totally bankrupt. In 1956 the American Medical Association called alcoholism a disease. The decision took a long time, but they had to be sure of their complete conclusion, namely, not only is alcoholism a disease but it is a terminal disease. In other words, if it is left untreated, the person dies.

The A.M.A. found, in their conclusions regarding alcohol, three major characteristics which are present in all terminal diseases. First, the disease is progressive, which means that it does not get better. There is no such thing as reversing the disease within you, which means that there is no way to *stop it.* The second is that, like other terminal diseases, alcoholism is a chronic disease. The individual is an alcoholic not because of too much drink the night before, but because he/she drank too much, too often, for that individual. The true alcoholic cannot touch alcohol at all. The third major characteristic is that there is a blind spot, which means the alcoholic is the last person to recognize what is going on in his or her life. An important note here regarding the foregoing: The people around the individual can readily see the deterioration that is occurring in each of the aforesaid areas, but the alcoholic cannot see it. That is why family members and significant people in the life of the patient are vital to the recovery process. They must understand that it is only by bringing together and educating these people so that they can confront the sick alcoholic with his/her deterioration that we can remove this blind spot and help the alcoholic see what is happening. "Tough love" — well named in this case — is called for here.

One last note: The budding alcoholic may have a very high tolerance for alcohol. He is the one who can drink them all under the table and still drive everyone home. Yes, for a while; but then he begins to need three quick drinks to start feeling good, to get up with the crowd. His tolerance for alcohol is going down. That is what this booklet is all about. It has been written for the one who answers these last lines by saying, "Who? Me? I'm no alley bum!" That's right—only five percent of alcoholics are on skid row. And you had better stop the soft guff about "having a drinking problem" and call it what it is—alcoholism.

Obsession

Alcoholics are described as obsessive in their attitude toward drink. Here is a fast picture of obsession, written by a bystander. "The man was just coming out of the anesthetic following serious abdominal surgery. The doctor was in the patient's room at the time. As the prostrate man's vision focused, he murmured, 'Doctor, tell me. Will I still be able to drink?'

"It would seem that most patients just returning from the door of death would ask questions like, 'How did the operation come out? What was the trouble inside? Was it cancer? How much of the intestine was taken out?' But not this fellow — he is an alcoholic. Evidently, no matter what they took out of him or left in him, he was still 'sick' — sick with the disease called alcoholism. I wonder how the wife and children felt when they heard this?"

Resentment

This describes what the "arrested" (never "cured") alcoholics have to live with for a long time, and they had better begin to work on it. In their minds, the failures were caused by someone else, never by themselves. They had begun their journey down the long, lonesome trail of alcoholism, angry at anyone who tried to suggest that drink was hurting them; and now that everything is out in the open they pretty well hate anyone and everyone who helped to turn on the floodlights. Those people cost them both their whiskey and their alibis. For a while, they will lie there and curse, feeling naked to their enemy's sword, but if they join A.A., an old timer will soon mark them: He knows what they are going through, and will know when to lance the wound and clean it so that the new pigeons (as they will be lovingly referred to by the clan) can live. Slowly, these new members will realize that their resentment was garbage; and one fine day, they may write some beautiful lines of thanks and of understanding to the ones they resented so deeply and to whose courage they owe, perhaps, their very lives.

The Slip

A slip is a return to alcohol. Let's talk about the A.A.'s desire to help alcoholics who have slipped. The point we would like to make is that going out to help others is not a chore to these people. Nor is it simply a tit-for-tat affair, that is, "Since somebody helped me; now I have the obligation of helping others."

No. It is all a matter of pain, pain that you went through. You simply cannot now sit still as another human being goes through it all alone while you have the words and the tools and the love to soften the pain, to help him or her start all over again. It is a strong conviction (and a practiced one) among the older Alcoholics Anonymous groups that if you do not run to help others, you are cutting yourself off from the branch, and you will die because you forgot or chose to forget that you are a life-carrier for the ones in pain, who, on their side, waited to exercise your love and make it flourish.

Notice the kind word "slipped" — not fell — just slipped. So get that balance back quickly — before the alcoholic hits the ground hard!

Arrested Alcoholism/Alcoholic

The alcoholic has a slight laugh, a very slight smile, for the double meaning of that word "arrested"; and, of course, it does not really infer any dealings with the law. To our sick friend it is a deadly serious word, because it is a continual reminder that there is no cure for alcoholism; there is only complete abstinence, by which we do not cure the disease but only arrest its progress, or, to put it more correctly, we arrest, we stop the symptoms — such as inefficiency, blackouts, etc. The disease is only held in balance within the victims. If they return to alcohol after even a long period of abstinence, they do not pick up the disease—as does one who is just starting his alcoholic trip—but, instead, pick it up at the point where they left it. Such persons sadly know the meaning of the word "arrested."